CBD for Dogs

Recue dog anxiety and Arthritis pain, Seizure Dog Epilepsy

JANINE WALBERGER

Copyright © 2019 Janine Walberger
All rights reserved.
ISBN: 9781656966797

Introduction

From pharmacies, pet stores, to even local gas stations. They're everywhere!

What are they?

Thanks to the high sales rate of Cannabidiol in the market and the speed at which its popularity increases daily, it is very obvious that this substance has come to write its name in the sands of time. Some countries, like the United States through the passage of the 2018 Farm Bill, have made the production of industrial hemp legal, and some states have also legalized recreational and medical cannabis, so that may also account for CBD's explosive popularity and availability.

But what seems to grow along with it among people is the confusion about what it is and what it is used for. If you are one of the people that seem to be seeing it everywhere but don't know what it is used for, you are not alone. You'll get acquainted with it as we go along.

Furthermore, people that have an idea of the power of CBD only relate it to human usage. They only know that CBD is used for treating chronic pain, epilepsy, insomnia, migraine, muscle spasms, nausea, Alzheimer's and Parkinson's diseases. But do they really know the power of CBD on pets, especially dogs?

Do you?

This is what this book hopes to address. In it, you will not only learn what CBD is all about and clear your doubt, but you will come to appreciate the effectiveness that comes with this potent substance especially on dogs. If your dog continuously showcases some undesirable symptoms, CBD can do the magic and restore it to its former glory.

If you are a dog owner, this should be exciting news for you.

Dogs are special and should be treated as such. There is nothing that beats the feeling of knowing that your dog is hale, hearty and doesn't have a care in the world.

Just like human beings, dogs (pets in general) can be saddled with problems that may either be self-induced or caused by illnesses. Because they do not have the ability to communicate effectively with people, they may tend to translate their pains and grievances through the noises they make.

On one or two occasions, we were too busy to listen. We have been saddled with our own problems and busy schedules that we do not prioritize the needs of the pets we own. We wake up in the morning, set out for work or school activities, probably head out to a few events thereafter and come home exhausted, not to mention the loads of domestic responsibilities that await us in our homes. What does the noise of our dogs have to do with anything?

We are all guilty of this.

But our dogs feel pain in ways that we can never imagine. They also have tendencies to convulse when their stomach becomes sensitive to foods they are not used to.

Can dogs get depressed? Oh yes, they can.

We will find out more about all these as we proceed.

So, shall we?

Chapter One: Introduction to CBD

What is CBD?

Here goes the almighty question. What really is CBD?

And we aren't just referring to the full meaning of CBD? What does CBD entail generally?

Let's have a look.

CBD is the short form for Cannabidiol. It is one of the 108 types of cannabinoids found in cannabis plants. The cannabis plant is a member of the Cannabaceae family, and although the number of this plant's species is unknown at the moment, three major species are widely recognized: Cannabis indica, Cannabis sativa, and Cannabis ruderalis (although cannabis ruderalis is usually mentioned under Cannabis sativa). It is worthy to note that cannabinoids are of two types- endocannabinoids, which are cannabinoids gotten from the body and phytocannabinoid which are gotten from plants. So, from this, you should already know where CBD falls in.

Yeah?

Good. Let's proceed.

The two major extracts of the cannabis plant are the Tetrahydrocannabinol (THC) and the Cannabidiol (CBD) which are gotten from Cannabis sativa and Cannabis indica in large quantities from their strains respectively. This doesn't mean that the other cannabis extract can't be extracted from the other plant species. It only means that they are present there in small quantities. For instance, CBD can be found in Cannabis Sativa but not as much as THC. Other types of cannabinoids include Tetrahydrocannabinolic acid (THCA), cannabinol (CBN), cannabigerol (CBG), cannabivarin (CBV), cannabidivarin (CBDV), cannabicyclol (CBL), and the rest of them.

I am sure you are probably thinking, "Since this plant is gotten from cannabis, won't I experience feelings of highness or dizziness? My dog needs to be active so it can't afford to take this right now if it would cause this effect!"

Happy to dissolve your fears, darling…

The beautiful thing about CBD is its non-psychoactive effect, so no matter how you take it, you or your dog cannot get high. Although some people complain of some sort of uneasiness when they take it for the first time because of the sensitivity of their bodies (some pets also react when they take it for the first time as well), there is nothing to be scared about with this. What you should fear is CBD's evil cousin, tetrahydrocannabinol (THC). Gotten in large quantity from cannabis Sativa, this is the substance that gives Cannabis plants a bad name in general. It is one of the major constituents of THC and it is what stimulates the pleasure hormones in the brain and causes a feeling of highness and dizziness when taken, which invariably leads to addiction among drug users. Some effects of THC include dizziness, bronchitis, reddened eyes, dysphoria, cough, ataxia, dryness of the mouth (which may lead to periodontitis), low sperm production, anxiety, reduced body coordination, tachycardia and worse of all, the pupils of the eye begin to respond slowly to light. This is why most people are not encouraged to take cannabis except on medicinal grounds, as it may cause blood pressure changes, increase the chances of getting angina, myocardial infarction, cardiomyopathy, ischemic attack, arrhythmias, stroke, and all these increase mortality rates.

How worse can it get?

However, we aren't saying that THC is completely bad, as research has shown that it is responsible for cannabis' many therapeutic effects, but it is advised that it is taken based on a doctor's prescription. Overdose or addiction could lead to the effects listed above.

Okay. Snap. Let us go back to our happy and ever joyful CBD.

Now you may also be thinking, "Why has this only been focusing on the effects of CBD on humans and not on dogs?"

It is very important that you note how the CBD works generally before you can understand its effect on pets. CBD provides all the amazing health benefits to human beings by attaching itself to the receptors (CB1 and CB2) in the endocannabinoid system of the human body. There, it plays a very huge role in regulating sleep and memory. In the same vein, CBD also plays a significant role in reducing anxiety, depression, chronic pain and stress in dogs.

How do you know when your dog is having any issue?

It's simple: Pay close attention. If you can't do it personally, tell a family member or friend to do it for you, or better still, hire someone. There is no gain in having a pet you do not take care of.

Dogs are very simple beings, so detecting issues with them is not supposed to be a herculean task. Most dogs relay their uncomfortable states by mostly growling if they are in pain when they meet an adversary or are in a situation that gets them afraid, and makes low pitiful noises and lie low when they are hungry or experiencing chronic pain. All you have to do is listen. The signs are there.

So, you may also be thinking, again, "Since CBD is mostly taken by humans, is it safe for my dog?"

This leads us to the next chapter

Chapter Two: Types of CBD and Safety Measures for your Dog

Now, we are going to look at safety from two angles- physical safety and legality.

Recall that we stated the origin of CBD in the previous chapter, where it was mentioned that CBD is one of the phytocannabinoid extracted from the cannabis plant. One of the main reasons why CBD has grown in popularity is its non-psychoactive effect despite being gotten from a cannabis plant. This implies that no matter the quantity in which it is taken, it generally does not cause any psychoactive effect, or what people term as 'being high'. So, you do not have to worry about your dog getting excessively high or acting all crazy. Everything is under control.

However, caution must be taken in this regard. Despite it being ascertained as generally safe, there have been some reports of side effects after usage which differs from person to person, although very rare. Some people experience a sense of drowsiness, tiredness, or slight stomach pains, diarrhea, but it quickly washes off with time. In the same vein, your dog may react with CBD if it has a very sensitive system by either feeling a bit drowsy or nauseous. Furthermore, research has shown that pregnant dogs should not take CBD for fear of side effects on the unborn, so you should take note. This is why it is always recommended that you have the veterinary doctor run a checkup on your dog to ascertain whether your dog can handle CBD ingestion or not. Never assume that CBD is okay for your dog at that moment, regardless of the situation. You may put your dog at risk of something it may never be able to recover from. Self-medication has never been the answer and will never be.

The truth is that there haven't been enough studies to prove the scientific authenticity of CBD on human beings and pets. Most of the claims are gotten from anecdotal evidence and testimonies from benefactors. But with the few ones that have been carried out, there hasn't been any cause for alarm, so your dog is safe. We all are.

Another thing you need to consider before giving your dog CBD is the drugs it is already on. Because of the chemical composition in these drugs, CBD can react with these drugs and produce undesirable effects on your dog. Most people give their dogs CBD with the hope that it will automatically heal them, even if the symptoms are way more complicated than they can handle. If your dog has issues and is already on some form of medication, it is advised that you allow it to finish the drugs, then book another appointment with the veterinary doctor to ascertain whether your dog is fine, needs another round of medication, needs more complicated procedures to be done on it or whether or not CBD should be administered. If the answer to the latter is no, it's best you take your dog home to rest. You weren't trained to be a vet, so don't try to be one.

Now, onto the legal part. Since industrial cannabis is unauthorized in several countries, getting CBD for your dog might be difficult. So, before you get one, the first thing you have to do asides consulting a veterinary doctor is to check whether cannabis is legal in your country. Using the United States as a case study, the passage of the 2018 Farm Bill act which has fully legalized hemp has enabled CBD to thrive. This law implies that consumers everywhere, as long as they comply with the laws of their state, can grow hemp at their convenience, and use hemp products which will include CBD. But that is federal law, so each state decides its policy. Some states like Alaska, Colorado, Maine, Massachusetts, Michigan, Oregon, Vermont, California, etc. have legalized both CBD and marijuana for recreational purposes. Some states have legalized it only for medicinal purposes. Some states have even legalized only CBD oil. While states like Nebraska, South Dakota, and Idaho have banned their production and use completely. So if you are staying in these states, it's best you stay out of trouble and avoid giving CBD to your dog. Always watch out for rules and try your best to avoid them, because people that respect law and order, and listen to good instruction and advice, tend to live long…

In summary, there are no serious side effects of CBD, except rare reports from people with very sensitive body systems. The main aim of Cannabidiol is to provide wellness and good health to humans and pets. So, allow your pet to enjoy the rich benefits CBD has to provide.

So, having established this, what is the best CBD spectrum to get for your dog?

Types Of CBD- Full Spectrum, Broad Spectrum and Isolate

Recall that in our previous chapters, we discussed what CBD is in general. It was stated that CBD stands for Cannabidiol, a phytocannabinoid that is gotten from the cannabis plant, and the beautiful thing about it is that it does not have a psychoactive effect on people and pets, that is, it doesn't cause what we generally term as highness, unlike THC. Tetrahydrocannabinol (THC) is more like an evil cousin to CBD as it causes highness when one takes marijuana. Note that THC and CBD are just two of the 108 different types of cannabinoids gotten from the cannabis plants. They are the major extracts.

It was also mentioned that because CBD has non-psychoactive effects, it is generally safe for use on your dog, except if it is on medication or has a sensitive system. So, it is recommended that you visit a veterinary doctor and get your dog checked before administering CBD on it. Then, the legality of a place also matters because some countries of the world haven't yet legalized industrial hemp, and some states of the countries still have rules that prohibit free usage, so you have to know the laws of your place before buying CBD

You must remember all these before we proceed.

So now you have decided to buy CBD for your dog. Good choice!

You majestically walk into a pet store, greet the receptionist and begin your selection. But you are finding CBD isolate on one corner, broad-spectrum CBD on another counter, full-spectrum CBD right in front of you… and you are like, "It's only CBD I came to buy. What's all this?"

Relax. You got this.

While all these names may look similar, they are not in any way. They are different types of CBD, each with its own uniqueness, so it is important that you understand them before buying. Note that the two major types are the full spectrum CBD and CBD isolate, but we will also look at the broad-spectrum CBD. So let's take a look, shall we?

CBD ISOLATE

No. This is not CBD that is kept in a corner of your bedroom, away from light and human (or pet) touch. It is just the purest form of CBD.

In science, the word 'isolate' usually refers to the purest form of a compound which is gotten by extracting that compound from its normal environment and completely isolating it from other compounds. In other words, CBD isolate is the purest form of CBD that is obtained by removing all other compounds seen in the cannabis plant which includes terpenes, flavonoids, etc. CBD isolate is usually extracted from hemp, because of its low THC content.

So the question now is, should you get this for your dog?

This book is here to spill undiluted truth, so here are the pros of using CBD on your dog:

- It is extremely safe: It is the safest form of CBD you will ever find since it is in its purest form and does not have any psychoactive effect.

- Your dog will not test positive for THC: If the need arises for your dog to be checked for THC, there is a very high chance that it will not test positive.

But you know that there are cons for every pro, right?

Your dog may not get the full benefits: Even though this is the purest form of CBD, your dog may not get the full benefits and privileges from other cannabinoids. For instance, if your dog has chronic pain, CBD isolate may not be able to do the trick because the substance only works in conjunction with THC. That is why THC is usually recommended and legalized for medicinal purposes only.

This also relates to illnesses that other cannabinoids can heal as well.

So, on what occasions should your dog be given CBD isolate?

- If the vet requests for your dog to take CBD in large quantity, then CBD isolate is probably your best bet

- If your dog is going to be tested for drugs, you should give it CBD isolate to avoid being questioned for traces of THC.

- If you are living in a state (or country as the case may be) with zero tolerance for THC, then you should give your dog CBD isolate.

- If you are giving your dog CBD for the first time and you are not sure how it is going to respond to you, it should start with CBD isolate.

Let's move over to full spectrum

FULL SPECTRUM CBD

This is the CBD whose extracts consist of all the compounds that are naturally found in the cannabis plant in their full form. This means that this CBD contains terpenes, flavonoids and other cannabinoids. Think of full-spectrum CBD as the opposite of CBD isolate.

What is the work of full spectrum CBD?

Because CBD is extracted with all the other compounds from the plant, the therapeutic and healing benefits of each of the cannabinoids are magnified. This is to say that your dog not only gets the benefits of CBD, but it gets those from other compounds as well. This is known as the Entourage effect

The Entourage effect is simply a mechanism whereby different cannabis compounds work together in synergy to regulate the total psychoactive effects of the cannabis plant, and this is controlled majorly by the THC.

Before, people generally believed that CBD isolate was more effective than full spectrum CBD because it was in his purest form. But research done in 2005 by the Lautenberg Center for General Tumor Immunology in Jerusalem has proven that belief to be incorrect. It showed that people who took full spectrum CBD had better reliefs than those who took CBD isolate. It also showed that the dosage of full spectrum was directly proportional to the effects produced (the higher the dosage, the higher the effects), with the effect of CBD remaining the same. So we are going to liken this experiment to dogs as well.

So what are the advantages of giving full spectrum CBD to your dogs?

- **Entourage effect**: As stated earlier, the entourage effect will play a significant role in helping your dog heal. They will be able to benefit from the other cannabinoids.

- **Fewer production processes**: Unlike the CBD isolate which is extracted from the cannabis plant and kept separate from other compounds, full spectrum CBD does not undergo all those processes, so production time is lessened.

- Of course, you cannot find an advantage without a disadvantage, right?

- **High psychoactive effect**: full spectrum CBD tends to have a high psychoactive effect on your dog. Since there is a combination of all the cannabinoids and they are working together, the effects of THC and other psychoactive compounds will come to play. Furthermore, recall that the entourage effect is largely regulated by the THC for all the therapeutic benefits to be given. So, if you do not want your dog acting all crazy, full spectrum CBD can take a seat.

- If you are living in a state with zero tolerance for THC, buying full spectrum CBD may pose legal problems for you.

- Your dog may be tested positive for THC.

So, on what occasions should one use full spectrum CBD?

- If cannabis is legal in your state, you can proceed with this

- If your dog has an illness that CBD isolate (or broad spectrum) cannot solve.

- If the vet requests that your dog takes a substance with a specific CBD to THC ratio, then the full spectrum is your best bet

BROAD SPECTRUM CBD

As stated earlier, the two major types of CBD are CBD isolate and full spectrum CBD, so broad spectrum CBD sort of combines the features of the two. Just like the full spectrum, the other compounds like the flavonoids, terpenes and the like are extracted with the CBD, but as the CBD isolate, THC is totally isolated.

This means that your dog can have the full benefits of all the other compounds without having to worry about the psychoactive effects of THC. The entourage effect is felt in full without getting high.

Isn't that amazing?

So, what are the pros?

- The entourage effect is felt: Dogs can get benefits from CBD and other compounds.

- It is very safe: Since THC is isolated from it, be assured that it is very safe for your dogs, except they are on other medications or are sensitive to CBD. There is no risk of psychoactive effects.

Wherever there is a pro, there is a con:

- Takes less research and production time: Just like the full spectrum CBD, it takes lesser time to produce since it is only THC that is extracted.

- It is not readily available: Since CBD isolate and broad-spectrum CBD are the major types in the market, broad spectrum CBDs are quite hard to find, even in pet stores. So, if you see one, count yourself lucky!

So, on what occasion should your dog take CBD?

- If your dog is taking CBD for the first time and you are scared of the psychoactive effects of THC, then broad spectrum CBD is probably the best option.

- Once again, if you are staying in a place with stringent THC laws, you can use this. Your dog won't test positive for THC.

- If your dog has an illness that CBD isolate cannot handle, instead of quickly resorting to full spectrum, it can take broad spectrum and see where it leads. But this must be under the guidance of a vet.

However, one thing you must note is that no one CBD supersedes the effects of the others. They are all different and each one has its own uniqueness and the problems it is meant to solve. All you have to do is note the symptoms your dog is having, consult a vet and choose a CBD that suits that problem.

Chapter Three: Benefits of CBD and How to Cope with the Side Effects, if Any

If you have gotten to this chapter of the book, Congratulations. You are almost halfway through the book. For the rest of the book, we will be showing you the benefits of CBD oil and treats for your dogs and how you can use them properly. CBD Oil comes with many benefits due to the contents laid out in the previous chapter. In this chapter, we will be giving you readers 7 strong benefits of CBD and why it is highly recommended, especially for Pets like Dogs.

1. It is a very powerful painkiller.

For so many years, the use of CBD has been very effective in the fight against pain in the body. Humans, over the years, have used CBD to cure a lot of ailments. CBD is used as a very strong painkiller and for pets like dogs, it is no different. Over the years, a lot of studies have been conducted and these studies have shown that CBD is a very great substance for killing the pain. Due to the antioxidant properties present in the CBD composition, it has great effects on the body of the dogs. These effects are anti-inflammatory, and it helps to improve stiffness. Another great thing that the use of CBD does to the body is that it has analgesic properties which helps the dogs to reduce the perception of pain present in the brain of the animal.

2. It is good antiemetic medicine.

There are a lot of cases where dogs have been seen in serious nauseating conditions. When they are in this condition, they are often prone to a lot of stress and vomiting. In most cases when these dogs experience this, it may often be a result of a certain unfavorable condition in which the dog may be facing. For the dog, this experience may not be very comfortable. It may lead to fatigue, weight loss and a decrease in the appetite of the dog. The use of CBD is a very effective cure in a situation like this. Scientific studies have shown that the use of CBD helps in stimulating the receptors responsible for anxiety. By the stimulation of these receptors, the feeling of nausea and vomiting will be greatly reduced. CBD is the best when it comes to this.

3. Proper enhancement of homeostasis.

For the readers who may not be familiar with the concept of homeostasis, we will try our best to break it down for you for proper understanding. Homeostasis is defined as the state of steady condition maintained by any physical and living organism. This state may be physical and chemical, and this state is dynamic and has several variables which are temperature and the balance of fluid. At equilibrium state, it is kept within certain limits which are known as the homeostatic state. It is simply described as the proper function of the human body and when all the bodily functions are in balance, this is when they occur to make sure that our body systems function optimally.

For Dogs, the use of CBD is very helpful in enhancing homeostasis. This is because it promotes the overall wellbeing of the pet.

4. It has good anti-inflammatory effects

Another reason why a lot of dog owners love using this CBD for dogs is because of its anti-inflammatory effects. CBD has very useful abilities. One of them is its ability to interact very well with the cells in the immune system. The Anti-inflammatory effects of CBD make it a very powerful substance used in the treatment of various harmful conditions.

When the CBD interacts with receptors in the dogs, it brings up a broad range of immune system responses. Among these responses is the ability to fight inflammation caused by the dis-functioning of the immune system. Once the CBD reduces the inflammation, all other conditions like pain, IBD, arthritis and more will be reduced. Always trust CBD Il and other CBD related products to give you the best results.

5. **It helps to reduce stress.**

It is important to note that pets like dogs also have issues, especially stress. The use of CBD on dogs help to effectively manage the presence of anxiety and stress that may occur in the dog. This stress could lead to a lot of anomalies which may bring a lot of harm to the dog. When a dog is stressed or anxious, there will be a lot of symptoms involved. These symptoms include; constant vomiting and barking, aggressive chewing, tremors, and constant urination.

The use of CBD in such cases like this have been known to reduce the feeling of stress and anxiety amongst dogs and help them feel better and more comfortable. How does it work? It works by targeting certain receptors present in the brain, thereby helping to reduce stress.

6. Prevents the growth of tumors in dogs.

On several occasions, there will be a presence of tumors spread throughout the body of the dog. If proper care is not taken, these tumors will eventually spread to most parts of the body causing a lot of irritation, discomfort and ill health. Tumors are very dangerous and the only way to get rid of them is to fight against them properly. Proper research has been done to show how effective CBD is in the fight against cancer and how it has worked properly.

In cases like this, what we need to do is to rely on CBD to prevent these tumors and protect our dogs from having such terrible experiences. The use of CBD is very useful in the fight against tumors because it has a lot of anticancer effects.

7. **Improves appetite**.

A dog needs to have a very healthy appetite. A healthy appetite makes the dogs more active and more useful as a pet in the family. Whenever a dog experiences a poor appetite, there will be a loss in the overall physical nature of the dog. The use of CBD is also very effective in helping these dogs regain their appetite back. The contents of the CBD increase appetite and when the appetite in the dogs are high, they will have a healthier look and feel.

In general, the use of CBD is very essential in the improvement of the overall health of the dog. As dog owners, the use of CBD should be included in all the diet plans giving to the dog. These pets are sensitive too and they should also be treated as important. It is very wrong to neglect them because when they are neglected medically, they are prone to a lot of physical and mental attacked. In the next sections of this book, we will be giving you readers a full breakdown of how CBD helps in reducing anxiety, curing arthritis and chronic seizure that may be happening to them.

Effects Of CBD

Recall in the previous chapter that we talked about the types of CBD. We have two major types of CBD which are the full spectrum CBD and the CBD isolate, then there is the broad-spectrum CBD which is a combination of the features of the two major ones.

The CBD isolate is the CBD that is isolated from all other compounds when extracted from the cannabis plant. The full spectrum is the CBD that is extracted with all other compounds like the terpenes, which creates the entourage effect. The compounds work together to magnify their individual effects, with THC playing a major role. Finally, we have the Broad-Spectrum CBD which consists of CBD and all other compounds except THC. This way, you don't have to worry about your dog going all crazy. It is important you note, however, that each type of CBD has its unique features and the problem it is meant to solve. The action of one does not supersede the other.

For instance, your dog may have an illness that requires large amounts of CBD, then it should go for CBD isolate. If it has an illness (usually one that involves physical pain) that requires some amount of THC, then full spectrum CBD may be the best option. But if it involves getting the entourage effects of all cannabinoids except THC, then the broad spectrum is your option. So, it all depends on what your dog needs.

Whether we like it or not, CBD is here to say. It is making such a huge round in the pet industry that a lot of veterinarians opt for it more than conventional medicine, even though they may be afraid to say it for fear of stringent THC laws. As you know, CBD is popular because of its effectiveness and non-psychoactive nature, so it is generally accepted as safe. CBD is used to treat several illnesses such as anxiety, depression, chronic pain, etc.

There has, however, been some rare reports about some mild side effects, and this is usually seen in sensitive dogs, dogs that are taking CBD for the first time or dogs that are on another medication.

WHAT ARE THESE EFFECTS?

- **Drowsiness**: As we mentioned earlier, CBD is used to treat anxiety and other mental illnesses, so for this reason, it is usually prescribed in high dosages. If your dog is unable to handle the effect, it might get drowsy, sleepy and let out low growls. If this persists, you need to pause the medication a bit.

- **Dryness** of mouth: Or you think dryness of mouth only affects humans? The mouths of dogs get dried once in a while, usually when they take high dosages of CBD because studies have shown that CBD can reduce the production of saliva when ingested. So, if you see your dog gulping down large amounts of water while on medication, know that CBD is at play.

- **Vomiting** and diarrhea: Your dog may also vomit and produce watery stool while on medication, especially if it is very sensitive to the food it takes. However, reports of this effect are very rare.

- **Dizziness**: This is one of the most popular but uncommon side effect of CBD in dogs, as they usually get lightheaded after taking it. One way to know if your dog is feeling dizzy is to watch its countenance closely. For instance, if you give your dog CBD, take it to an open show 20 minutes later and find it lying under a car or a bench, know that the CBD is beginning to take effect. But this hardly happens.

- **Low blood pressure**: This is another popular side effect of CBD, even among humans. High dosages of CBD are known to reduce blood pressure, which invariably leads to lightheadedness.

In general, these effects are very mild, and they tend to go away when the CBD has taken full effect in their bodies. The most important thing you have to do is to talk to a vet before administering CBD to your dog and be mindful of the medications it has been on (or is currently on) before administering it, as it could interact negatively with it.

So, what do you do when your dog starts experiencing these side effects?

As mentioned earlier, your dog can experience any of the side effects above, regardless of age or breed. It doesn't matter if you are giving your dog a chew-capsule or CBD oil. You have to monitor your dog's actions and behaviors closely. Once you start seeing these signs, it is advised that you stop administering the substance immediately. High dosages of CBD usually result in these effects, and they clear out once the CBD has diffused into the body system completely.

When these effects have worn out, it is also recommended that you restart with a lower dose, and watch again. If this dose is consistently given and the dog doesn't exhibit any side effect, you may then gradually increase the dosage until you have seen the desired result. But if these side effects persist, you need to visit the vet.

Another thing to note is that if you and your vet decide to get CBD for your dog, you must always go for high-quality products in whatever form (more on this later on) if you want to achieve the desired effect. Here are some quick tips:

a. Purchase organic products: The best CBD to buy is the organic one, and even if you are unable to buy it, you should at least get one that's free from pesticides, solvents, chemicals or other harmful chemicals.

b. Do not go for inferior products because of the price: You would always have an excuse to buy something of low quality because of the price. The economy is down. It isn't the first time. You need money to buy other important things like sneakers and movie tickets. We all do. But what is more important than taking care of your pet? Do not buy inferior products because of price because when the quality is top-notch, the prices increase.

c. Look at the analysis carefully: When you take your dog to the vet and he/she allows you to administer CBD on it, they usually tell you what type of CBD to buy. So, you have to look at the specifications on the literature that comes that with the substance. Find out whether it is CBD isolate, full or broad spectrum by looking at their CBD to THC ratio. You also have to note the quantity of CBD in these products, as most of them aren't what they appear to be.

d. Buy ones that are approved by the drug regulating agency of your country: As mentioned earlier, some countries have zero tolerance for marijuana and industrial hemp. Even if they permit, they would definitely have laws that regulate production and usage. Any CBD product that doesn't have any form of registration identity was either produced through the wrong means or didn't meet up the standards set by the agency. Buying them is a recipe for disaster. Ensure that you buy products that are registered and approved by the food and drug agency of your country.

When all these are done, half of your problems are solved.

Still, have doubts? You should not. It can transform your life in ways that you would never expect.

Chapter Four: How your Dog can Benefit from CBD- Anxiety

While in the production of this book, a friend of mine came to me and asked, do dogs also experience anxiety? I said yes. Dogs are also mammals just like human beings and they are also prone to having feelings of anxiety once in a while. For the readers of this book, who may not fully understand what anxiety is, we will do well to break it down for you.

Anxiety is described as your body's response to stressful activities. In a lot of cases, it may be very normal. In other cases, it may be due to a certain health condition of some sort. When they are caused by these health conditions, they are known as anxiety disorders.

Anxiety disorders seriously interfere with everyday life. Even the lives of the dogs in questions. They have a lot of terrible experiences and they will always find it difficult to live their lives comfortably. For these dogs, it will bring them a whole lot of discomfort.

The symptoms of anxiety in dogs are often very common and they are easily observed and noticed. These symptoms include. Restlessness and persistent barking, regular irritation and constant difficulty in movement. For dogs, it could lead to a whole lot of disaster.

Causes of Anxiety in Dogs.

- Phobia.

It is one of the major causes of fear in dogs, it is a very terrible experience when cannot get away or get through a terrible condition.

- Aging.

Dogs can also be anxious due to aging as well and it is a very common phenomenon. Aging is a result of a change in the nervous system in the body.

As a dog owner, you should always be able to detect when your dog is experiencing anxiety and anxiety-related disorders. Visit a veterinary behaviorist to check the behavior of your dog and know what to do whenever they need to do so.

HOW DO WE TAKE CARE OF THIS?

CBD is the right answer. CBD has been one of the major remedies in the treatment of anxiety and anxiety-related disorders. The National Institute of Drug Abuse, Maryland, United States of America has shown strong evidence that the use of CBD significantly reduces stress in animals such as dogs. By conducting several tests, they were able to show that in the dogs, a significant reduction in the heart rate was observed. When it comes to cases involving anxiety disorders, all the tests conducted have been proven positive.

Veterinary doctors all over the world strongly recommend the use of CBD for your dog. In several cases, people confuse the use of CBD to marijuana because they all come from the same source. They are different. The major difference between them is that CBD does not make the dog high.

HOW DOES CBD WORK TO REDUCE ANXIETY?

The major function of the CBD Oil is to interact with the endocannabinoid system. Proper interaction will enable the soothing of the body system which helps to alleviate anxiety.

In the body of the dog, the endocannabinoid system is described as a complex system in the body. The body possesses several CBD receptors spread throughout all the organs, the brain and in the central nervous system. These receptors are what is known as the endocannabinoid system, and when the body releases endocannabinoid substances, they interact with the natural receptors in the body and improves the body's natural ability to produce a mood stabilizer known as serotonin.

It is important to note that when giving your dog a dose of the CBD oil, it is better to start slowly and in smaller quantities. This is because CBD oils are very potent, and an overdose could lead to another thing in the body of the dog. Always ensure that you start the dose slowly and gradually increase it. This is to ensure that the amount of CBD intake present in the body will be controlled.

The actual CBD intake that the dog will require is solely dependent on two things. The first is the size of your dog. And the second is the potency of the CBD oil product you decide to go with. If your dog is very large, you may want to consider giving it more doses of the CBD oil. If the dog is well below 25lbs, the maximum amount that would be required for the dog is 600mg.

When selecting the right kind of product for your dog, there are a lot of questions that you may need to ask. Some of those questions include;

•**How is it tested?**

It is very important to know how your product is tested before you go ahead to purchase the drug.

- **What is the level of THC present in the substance?**

It is also very important to know the amount of THC present in the substance. Most manufacturers often care less about certain things like this. Then go ahead and create CBD products from plants that have high CBD content thereby causing havoc to the dogs. While checking for the THC content present in the chemical, you should know that the amount of THC that is ideal in this case is always less than 0.03%.

- Its organic nature: This is by far one of the most important things that you should always look out for when buying this product. Good CBD products are always made from hemp that is organically grown and process using pharma-grade ethanol. Always note this.

All these and much more which we could outline in this book are the important questions you need to ask your retailer or supplier before you proceed in buying these products. It is very important so you would not proceed to buy counterfeit products.

As a dog owner, you should not expect your dog to immediately become relieved and start going about routine activities. Most dogs show immediate response to the CBD treatment. Others take quite a long period to respond to this. What you need to do is to take your time and study the dog, give it the proper dosage and ensure that you monitor its response to the treatment.

Chapter Five: How your Dog can Benefit from CBD- Arthritis, and Epilepsy

We are very sure that at this point in the book, you have gotten some good knowledge and tips on how to properly take care of your pet when it is facing anxiety and anxiety-related disorders. You may be wondering how to treat your dog when it comes to arthritis.

When a dog gets arthritis, things could get very messy if it is not properly controlled. For the readers who do not have an idea of arthritis, we will give you the complete breakdown that you will need.

Arthritis is simply described as joint inflammation, and it can be a very painful experience. It can be caused by a lot of symptoms and for a dog, it can seriously affect regular movements. Common symptoms of arthritis include severe pain, stiffness of the affected area, and pain. If it is not properly treated, it could cause a serious amount of damage.

In most cases, the pain felt from suffering arthritis may be mild, in some cases, it may be severe. If they are not properly treated, it could remain there for years and get worse over time. Serious arthritis may lead to permanent and serious changes to the joint and in some cases, may only be seen on an x-ray.

For dogs, arthritis could lead to a lot of problems. In the United States, there is an estimated number of over 20 million dogs that are currently battling with arthritis. Among dogs, there is a very common type of arthritis known as osteoarthritis. It is caused by the reduction of the cartilage generation in the joint.

CAUSES FOR ARTHRITIS IN DOGS

Infection in the Joint

When there is an infection in the joint, it could lead to several problems around that area. The infection can be strong enough to damage the whole joint which could lead to arthritis.

Ligament Injury

An Injury in the ligament could be very terrible, especially for your dog. Ligament injuries are one of the major causes of arthritis in pets and the worst of them all is the cranial ligament tear. When the ligament is damaged, it could lead to a lot of problems and cause a lot of instability around that area.

Cartilage tear

This is also another way in which dogs could have arthritis and related issues. This can be found in dogs that are of a larger breed and can be caused by excessive feeding.

The cartilage is flexible, and it is referred to as a firm joint. At certain times, it may deteriorate i.e. collide against each other and cause stiffness. Osteoarthritis is caused due to the wearing off of the joint leading to a lot of problems and it mostly affects older dogs.

When a dog is suffering from arthritis, they are prone to be very inactive. The weight of your dog is very one of the major contributors when it comes to arthritis. If your dog is overweight, the tendency for your dog to suffer from arthritis would be very high. As part of the preventive measures, always ensure that your dog always goes through proper exercise.

HOW DOES CBD WORK TO PREVENT ARTHRITIS?

A lot of research conducted has shown that CBD stands to be one of the most effective treatments when it comes to Arthritis. It is very powerful because of its anti-inflammatory effects. CBD is a very safe substance that stands out to be very safe and less psychoactive. CBD has been tested a lot by various researchers worldwide and the substance is seen to have a better effect than other medications.

Just as earlier stated, when the CBD is consumed, it interacts with the endocannabinoid system present in the body. This system has receptors found in the brain and several parts of the body, When the CBD interacts with these receptors, its anti-inflammatory effects are produced. As a dog owner, there are certain things you need to keep in mind when you decide to treat your dog with CBD. Dogs are more sensitive when it comes to the reception of cannabinoids than other mammal species. Because of this, you have to always give dogs smaller doses than humans.

You must give your dog the right dose of the drug at all times. However, because of how the drug was made, it is incapable of causing an overdose. It is still advised that a proper structure should be used to administer this CBD oil in the dog. When you decide to give this dog in dosage, the doses should depend on the condition of the dog. The ideal dosage should be at least 2 times daily regularly.

Giving proper dosage is what you need to learn as a dog owner. However, it is important to note that before you proceed to give your dog this CBD treatment, you have to consult a veterinary doctor to know the right steps to take. A veterinary doctor will teach you what you need to do to properly treat your dog.

However, with all this said, the most important you also need to consider is the strength of the product. Most people need to know the contents of the products they decide to buy before they proceed to buy these products. Ensure that you are buying from a duly registered and licensed manufacturer and ensure that you have proper knowledge of the content. Always know what your dog prefers. Either the CBD in capsule form, oil or treats, this CBD can be infused into the dogs depending solely on what the dog prefers.

In summary, the use of CBD is highly recommended. Most CBD products are designed for mobility issues. There are a lot of products out there that are specially designed for the treatment of mobility issues. If you do not have a dog, but you are planning on getting one, I strongly believe that the details outlined in this book would help you to know what to do whenever you need to do it. Dogs are very precious creatures and at all times, they should be treated as such. Once you give your undivided attention in taking care of your dog, your dog will respond to you in a lot of great ways, more than you know.

Next, we will be discussing on CBD for Epilepsy and Seizures in Dogs. Yes, I am sure that at this point, you are very surprised. Dogs also experience epilepsy and seizures due to certain conditions they may be facing. In the next section, you will learn how to use CBD to Epilepsy and certain seizures that may happen to the dog. At this point, you should know the right approach when you just in case you begin to experience certain issues like this.

CBD FOR EPILEPSY AND SEIZURES

In some cases, your dogs may begin to experience some sort of seizures that you may not understand. A lot of dog owners we have had contact with have stated that these seizures often come at unexpected times and they often throw these dog owners off balance. As a dog owner, it is a very terrible experience when you have to see your dog going throw a very terrible experience that you have little or no experience in how to handle it. A typical seizure in a dog may be very small and subtle. Symptoms of seizures may include jerky feeling, heavy breaths, careless whining and a weak appearance. Serious seizures and epilepsy may lead to tremors, distress and even unconsciousness.

How are these seizures caused? Seizures are normally caused by an anomaly in the firing of the neurons present in the brain. As a dog owner, you do not have to hesitate to visit the veterinary doctor when your dog is experiencing seizures whether it is mild, or it is serious.

How do you deal with this?

When you are thinking of a natural remedy, CBD oil is the best and should be the only option. Just as we have earlier stated, CBD comes from the Cannabis plants and it is said to have good anti-convulsing effects. Due to the way this product is created, it will have no effects on the dog.

How does it work?

As earlier explained, the dog's internal system is made up of several receptors which are known as the endocannabinoid system. These receptors are very important, and they regulate the functions of the body. The endocannabinoid system maintains homeostasis by the synthesis in a stable environment. The mechanisms in the internal parts of the body lag when the seizure interacts with homeostasis.

In the body of the dog, the CB1 receptor is present in the nervous system, the brain, and the glands while the CB2 receptors are mainly in the part of the immune system. These two receptors are the major components of the endocannabinoid system. The CB1 receptors are the major receptors that are in charge of calming down the super-active neurons and take control of seizures. The CB1 supplements work with the two receptors but act better with the CB1 receptor. CBD is also very effective in the restoration of homeostasis in the body.

How effective is the CBD?

There are a lot of great effects that CBD has when dealing with the treatment of seizures. A lot of dog owners all over the world have commented greatly on the good effects the use of CBD has given to their pets. They have stated that these CBD products have saved their dogs from attacks and seizures that could have been very fatal. Researchers all over the world have done their very best when it comes to finding out the effectiveness of the product. So far, research has shown that over 89% of the dogs that have received CBD over the years have experienced a reduction in the seizures.

Chapter Six: Practical Ways to Treat your Dog with CBD

As you have come this far in this book, you may be wondering, how do we treat our pets with this product and make them comfortable?

Here is your answer.

To reduce seizures and frequent epileptic attacks on your dogs, you have to give them the CBD regularly. In an ideal situation, the best way to do it is to give your pet at least twice every day. As a dog owner, you should know by now that you should not do anything concerning medication without proper consultation and guidance from your veterinary doctor. Whatever your doctor prescribes for you, you must try them out and experiment with others to determine which product is more suitable for your dog. However, it is important to bear in mind that your dog cannot overdose from the drug, but it is still important to find the right amount and know the right way to give.

The CBD products are all in a wide range. Different products for different kinds of people and animals. It is now left for you to figure out how which one is right. CBD for dogs comes in various forms. It can also be given in various ways too. Either by extracting from a bottle and feeding the dog with a dropper to the mouth, giving the dog through the food it is given, rubbed n the skin of the dog or dropped on the paw for them to lick it themselves. Several ways are that are very effective when it comes to giving these CBD products. There are also a lot of CBD biscuits made by different manufacturers all over the world. There are also honey capsules and CBD ointments that can be used on the pet.

Before buying the products, you have to ensure that the product is well tested. Yes. This is very important. As a dog owner, you must not buy any product without having good knowledge of the organic content of the product. That is why your veterinary doctors are there for you. Before you walk into a store or a pharmacy to buy these products, ensure that you have good knowledge of the content you are looking for. Do not go about buying products that you have little or no idea about. A good CBD product has the following features.

1. Highly potent.

2. Less than 0.3% THC content present in the substance.

3. It is a non-psychoactive product.

4. It is extracted using only water and food-grade ethanol.

5. The cannabis is grown and harvested using organic methods only.

These specifications are the ideal specifications that are needed when you are on the lookout for a good and potent CBD product. However, just as I have stated in the previous parts of this book, your veterinary doctor is the most important person in cases like this. In most cases, your dog may require a higher dose of medicine. Only your vet will tell you this.

The Bottom line.

CBD Oil has made a lot of lives easier over the years. The contents of these substances have helped a lot of lives become well and for pets, they are no different. In the marketplace today, CBD products stand out as one of the best in curing various physical and mental ailments in the body. Several hospitals, health centers, and therapeutic facilities have recommended the use of these products, especially for dogs.

Dogs are very lovely and lively creatures and regularly, they need to be taken care of. When proper treatment and proper care is given to these animals, it will put them in a condition that will be favorable for you. As a dog owner reading this book, you have seen the reason why the use of CBD is very crucial for taking care of your dog. If you are yet to do so, quickly rush down to the nearest veterinary doctor and seek proper guidance and counsel on how you can make good use of this product for your dog. Throughout the whole process of administering this CBD on your dog, never neglect the instructions of your vet because they are the once that know better when it comes to cases like this.

Conclusion

Dear readers, you know all about CBD for dogs and how to use them for the best purposes. The use of CBD has been scientifically proven to be very effective at curbing a lot of problems in the body of mammals. It has been testing and proven effective for humans, now, we have shown you in this book that it will also have a very positive effect on dogs.

For the readers of this book who do not have any idea of what CBD is all about, the first chapter of this book has given you a very concrete breakdown. We have explained the organic composition of CBD and how it works to relieve the entire body system. Is CBD Safe? WE have answered all those questions for you. In this book, a proper explanation of the safety of CBD was shown to tell you that you should not be afraid or worried when administering this product.

Full Spectrum and Isolate are the two main types of CBD that you should be looking out for when it comes to the treatment of your dog. As a dog owner, you should know the kind of CBD products and types you should administer to your dog for full effect.

In case you are having doubts about the efficiency of the product, the effects of the CBD products have also been given to you. It is very important to note that although CBD products are gotten from the Hemp plant, it is very safe. A good CBD product will not get your dog high under any circumstance. Before you go out to purchase these CBD products, always ensure that you purchase the right one.

There are three main types of ailments that a dog may experience. Anxiety, arthritis, and seizure. However, these three ailments can be treated with the use of CBD. The first ailment is anxiety. Anxiety is a very serious problem that occurs in a lot of dogs. We have shown you the causes and effects of anxiety and anxiety-related disorders in dogs and how the use of CBD stands out to be very effective. A complete breakdown of all you need to effectively treat these problems has been given to you in this book.

We also discussed arthritis. This is a very serious ailment and just like the way it happens in humans, it also occurs in the same way for dogs. In the earlier chapter of this book, we have shown you the various causes of arthritis in dogs and its various effects. Since we are discussing CBD, we also mentioned how CBD stands out as a very effective treatment for arthritis and other related ailments.

Seizures occur almost as often as other ailments mentioned and, in most cases, it is the most dangerous. Its causes and effects have also mentioned and how it can also be treated with CBD.